FREE MEDICINE

6 SUPER POWERFUL SIMPLE HEALTH YOGA TECHNIQUES

I0440126

A PRACTICAL GUIDE TO HEALTH AND WELLNESS

- A step-by-step guide
- Practical yoga, based on personal experiences
- Easy exercises that motivate everyone

GRACE PRABHA

First published 2023

Copyright © 2023 GRACE PRABHA

This publication is designed to provide accurate and authoritative information in regard to the subject matter covered. It is sold with the understanding that neither the author nor the publisher is engaged in rendering legal, investment, accounting, or other professional services. While the publisher and author have used their best efforts in preparing this book, they make no representations or warranties concerning the accuracy or completeness of the book's contents and specifically disclaim any implied warranties of merchantability or fitness for a particular purpose. No warranty may be created or extended by sales representatives or written sales materials.

Script Editor: Mr.Faris Abdelbasit

Contents

Disclaimer

It is recommended that you seek advice from a medical professional before starting any fitness program, including this one, to ensure that it suits your individual needs. This is especially important if you have a history of heart disease or high blood pressure, or if you have experienced chest pain in the past.

If you experience any discomfort that could pose a threat while exercising, stop immediately and consult a healthcare professional before resuming. If you choose to use any information from this book for personal use, which is your constitutional right, the author assumes no responsibility for your actions.

I INTRODUCTION

"Take care of your body. It's the
only place you have to live."

- Emanuel James Rohn

"Health is Wealth". We all acknowledge the value of good health in our present era of AI and bot technologies. Numerous options, such as traditional yoga, meditation, and modern fitness programs, are at our disposal to improve physical and mental wellness. I am sure that we have all experimented with some of them, only to abandon them later. Even after attending some of the finest programs during these trials, there may be instances when sustaining long-term commitment proves challenging, even with the help of the most exceptional tools tested daily. Nevertheless, our minds, perpetually acting like children, wish to do more to keep us fit, healthy, and content.

As a practitioner of alternative medicine, I consistently recommend certain exercises and yoga poses as part of my therapy programs or offer them as a free guide to people I meet. They are very excited to see the results and give positive feedback with delight. You see, as always, drugless practices require a continuous commitment to keep us healthy. I advise following these practices for a couple of months to experience the benefits. My friends say "Sure," but it does not become part of their daily routine.

Whenever I inquire about their exercise progress in subsequent meetings, they reply, "Well, you see, with so many priorities in my daily routine, I cannot even eat on time, let alone find time for the exercises."

Hearing this kind of reply very often, my thoughts turned toward finding some simple yet effective yoga movements to keep people in good health. Should I not show my acquaintances a workable, healthy path? After all, it is my passion to help and to heal!

There are several proven reasons why people struggle to continue a regular workout routine.

* Busy schedules (what could possibly be more important than our health?)

* Less priority is given to health (Not such a great mindset.)

* Not a conducive environment at home (limited space or too many people around.)

* Decreasing motivation day by day (this needs to be addressed.)

* There are numerous workouts, which demand significant time and effort (let's learn the efficient ones.)

* Not finding the right trainer (understandable.)

* Some health issues hindering workout schedules (definitely requires attention.)

* Lack of awareness about simple workouts. (Not possible after reading this book!)

Who most often finds themselves in the above situations, becoming less inclined towards workouts?

In my observations, they are primarily mothers, whether they be homemakers or working professionals. Mums are multi-taskers and incomparable human beings—my constant salute goes to them.

These amazing ladies might overlook carving out 15 to 20 minutes for personal yoga or similar activities. Why? Because they always prioritize doing something for their loved ones over themselves.

Secondly, businesspeople, driven by the constant pursuit of enhancing their income, feel certain that everything else in their lives is less important. Their aims are primarily focused on profits, leaving little room for their healthcare practices.

Finally, my beloved students find themselves in a similar predicament. With a barrage of term tests, board exams, and daily assessments, the focus of today's students is diverted from embracing a healthy lifestyle. Timidly entangled in the pursuit of high grades, academic commitments tightly bind their schedules. They have little time even to notice the people around them. The realm of mobile phones attracts their attention, leaving very little time for self-care.

Whatever the reasons, skipping the crucial workouts for the well-being of our body and mind is not a wise idea.

Throughout your journey of exploration and research, many of you have likely come across a multitude of exercises and workout routines, each contributing to your well-being in various ways. However, I'm sure you would agree that knowing a handful of potent exercise techniques can prove invaluable on many occasions. This book introduces yoga exercises that are not only potent but also easy to perform within a short time frame.

This exercise program is a culmination of the author's 21 years of experience in yoga and various other workout practices. Throughout this period, like many, I found myself making excuses for skipping my daily workouts. Then, one day, out of the blue, I had an epiphany – excuses needed to be discarded to strike the right balance between body and mind activities alongside my regular routines. This prompted me to select a few exercises, incorporate them seamlessly into my routine, and share them with my associates. Analysing the results carefully yielded impressive outcomes. Today, I am delighted to share these exercises with a global audience.

My Journey

I embarked on my yoga journey with Simple Kundalini Yoga (SKY) well before completing my undergraduate studies. All was going well until marriage brought about changes – relocating to a new place, new projects at work, and more. Then, the kids were born. Conventional beliefs suggested refraining from intense workouts after two consecutive caesareans, making it challenging to find time for myself. I completely stopped any health exercises, and everything seemed fine for a while. Unexpectedly, after a few miles of walking one day, back pain struck. It served as a reminder of my forgotten yoga routine. That's when I decided to join a yoga class, managing to squeeze it into my schedule.

One fine day, while playing with my kids, attempting to get up resulted in a spine-cracking sound, audible only to my consciousness as I fell unconscious. All I could tell myself was, "Breathe! Everything will be fine. Just keep breathing." After a couple of minutes, I regained my senses, feeling excruciating pain in the lumbar area. I could hardly move my legs. It was a paralysis attack, and I found myself bedridden for a month, facing lumbar region degeneration. My energy levels varied each day, and it was a time of self-enlightenment. I was fully immersed in the present moment – and all for the better! It marked the realization of the "Health is Wealth" moment, a triumphant moment of enlightenment.

My recovery was possible through consistent efforts, supported by yoga, acupuncture, Dorn therapy, and homeopathic treatments. Dr. Mahalakshmi played a pivotal role, assisting me in every aspect of my revival. She guided me to my hobbies and happiness. With her guidance, I resumed my usual yoga course and other exercises after a year-long gap.

Since then, I've delved into learning numerous exercises, therapies, and meditation techniques. As I returned to normalcy, I resumed my regular duties and responsibilities. Concurrently, I enrolled in an alternative medicine and therapy course to become a professional in the field. I've embraced a sustainable lifestyle, respecting Mother Nature in her way. However, time management became a challenge in my schedule. Allocating one hour for exercise seemed like a significant time investment, a sentiment echoed by my associates.

It was as if I needed to invent a time manager! Armed with the knowledge of various techniques, I initiated my research, focusing on the uniqueness, differences, and integrations of these methods. Over time, I identified specific exercises that contribute significantly to our health, laying the foundation for this comprehensive health program.

In the realm of therapy, the body is viewed holistically, and there is no disconnection based on specific diseases. Disease names and descriptions often instil more fear in us than the actual impact of the disease on us. Hence, throughout this book, I approach yoga techniques from a holistic and health-oriented perspective rather than associating them with disease correction.

This book serves as a roadmap, guiding you on how to seamlessly integrate powerful and straightforward exercises into your daily life, enabling you to lead a healthy and balanced life without the need for an extensively long workout routine. Now, doesn't that sound appealing?

II OVERVIEW OF SPS HEALTH YOGA TECHNIQUES

"Your health account and bank account are the same thing. The more you put in, the more you can take out."

- Francois Henri LaLanne

As I mentioned earlier, through my extensive research, I have identified six exercises or yoga techniques that stand out as particularly potent and beneficial for both physical and mental well-being. These techniques are collectively referred to as SPS Yoga, where SPS stands for Super-Powerful-Simple.

Having shared these techniques with many individuals, I have witnessed beneficial results. These exercises are combinations of various yoga poses and practices that I have learned over many years, and their effectiveness has been validated by numerous people I know.

Who can do these exercises?

These are simple yoga techniques designed to be accessible to individuals of all ages, from a two-year-old child to seniors. Age is just a number, and with these exercises, this statement certainly holds true.

Explore these methods as natural wellness solutions accessible to all, inviting everyone to engage and revel in their benefits

While they are suitable for individuals of any age, I particularly dedicate these practices to:

* Anyone unable to do conventional yoga or workouts due to time constraints;

* Those who embrace minimalism, seeking maximum health benefits with minimal effort and resources.

* Individuals looking for a quick yet comprehensive workout that seamlessly fits into their busy daily schedules.

Highlights of this program:

* Just six exercises, which can be done individually or as a complete set;

* They should be performed every day, or every few days, or along with other workouts as and when needed;

* Feel free to adjust the sequence of exercises based on your preferences for time, effort, and desired results.

The exercises are simple but impactful. This program is based on the idea that repeating a small number of practices regularly can significantly change how we think about fitness and exercise.

This program focuses on a few foundational exercises, each emphasizing an essential human movement pattern. The human body is naturally designed for these organic movements, and practising them regularly with minimal effort can yield significant and lasting benefits. Consistent conscious practice of each exercise can contribute to the development of robust, symmetrical, and functionally stable physical and mental well-being.

Essentials

* Keep a joyful smile on your face throughout these exercises!

"Illuminate your face with a smile to spread happiness all

around you."

* *Observe yourself while doing these workouts*. Be mindful of what you are doing. Often, our bodies are physically present, but our minds wander elsewhere.

"Observing our actions helps anchor our thoughts in the present."

* *Be yourself*. Allow your inner child to act. Our bodies and minds are closely tied to our desires and preferences. So be flexible, and listen to them.

"Yoga is best enjoyed with your 'unrestricted mode' turned ON."

I once had a friend whose son, during his undergraduate studies, mentioned that he occasionally enjoyed sleeping in the rabbit pose (sitting on folded legs and bending forward in a prayer pose). If that resonates with you, go ahead. Follow your heart and honour your desires.

* *Slower is better*. Performing these exercises as slowly as possible yields better results. Even if the number of "reps" is limited, taking the time to perform them mindfully provides more benefits. Moving slowly keeps the mind engaged. Otherwise, your thoughts may drift elsewhere, and you end up merely moving your body parts (which isn't exercise).

Each yoga technique, whether in part or in full, is a feast for both the body and mind. Give it its due importance in a holistic manner. Grasping its blueprint contributes significantly to physical and mental well-being.

III EXERCISE 1: STRETCHING AND BENDING

"To keep the body in good health is a duty... otherwise, we shall not be able to keep our mind strong and clear."

\-   Lord Buddha

Our body requires ample stretching and bending to maintain the health of our muscles and joints. This stimulates the blood supply and promotes the healthy functioning of our lymphatic system.

Technique:

This exercise is a combination of the following:

- Urdhva hastasana,
- Padahastasana, and
- Jalandara Bandha.

Directions:

- Do this exercise as soon as you step out of bed.
- Afterward, it can be done at any time of the day when refreshment is needed.
- While doing this exercise, thank Mother Earth for her blessings and care for you.

Execution of steps:

Step 1. Urdhva Hastasana / Raised Hand Pose

This pose emphasizes alignment, teaching us to align from the base up to the sky, both externally and internally. Focus on feeling inward and turn your awareness to your body.

➢ **Stand straight with your** feet shoulder-width apart.

➢ **Let your feet connect with the earth** through your big toes, heels, and the edges of your feet.

➢ **Gently stretch your chest upwards** and

➢ **Draw your shoulders back.**

➢ **Raise your arms over your head.**

➢ **Keep your hands up** with your palms facing each other in a prayer pose.

➢ **Keep your arms straight, gently look up,** directing your gaze towards your thumbs.

➢ **Stay in this position for a few seconds** before proceeding to the next step.

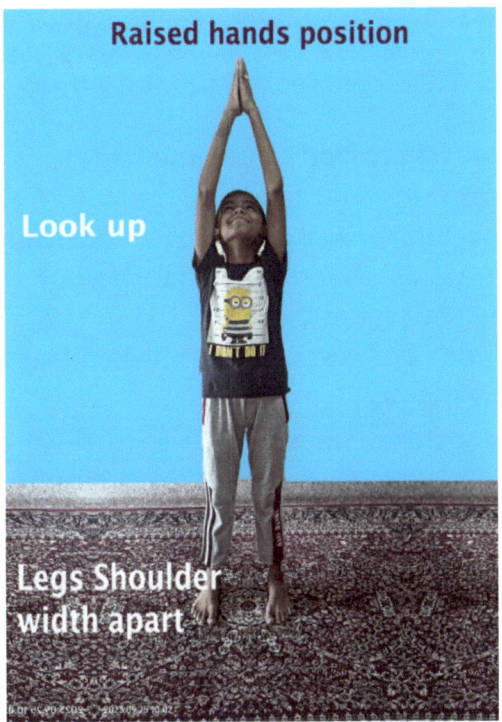

Picture 1: Stretching / Raised Hands position

Step 2. Pathahastasana / Forward Bend

This pose balances our position at the Nabhi (navel point) and brings alignment. This is the most essential pose of many therapies.

> From step 1, **bring your body forward and bend down.**

> **Pull your shoulders and hands forward** towards the floor.

> **Turn your head down** and bring your chin down to touch the top of your chest.

> **Bring your hands** down to touch the big toes or ground.

> Stay in this position for a few seconds.

Note: Be aware of your body limits. Stretch your body to its maximum flexibility gradually every day, aiming to bend down to touch the floor.

Dos:

- ✓ Be present with your body movements.
- ✓ Keep a big smile on your face.
- ✓ Gradually stretch to reach this perfect position.
- ✓ Bend your knees slightly to balance your weight while raising your hands.
- ✓ Try to keep your knees straight while bending down to stretch the nerves.
- ✓ Repeat at least three times, and up to nine times.

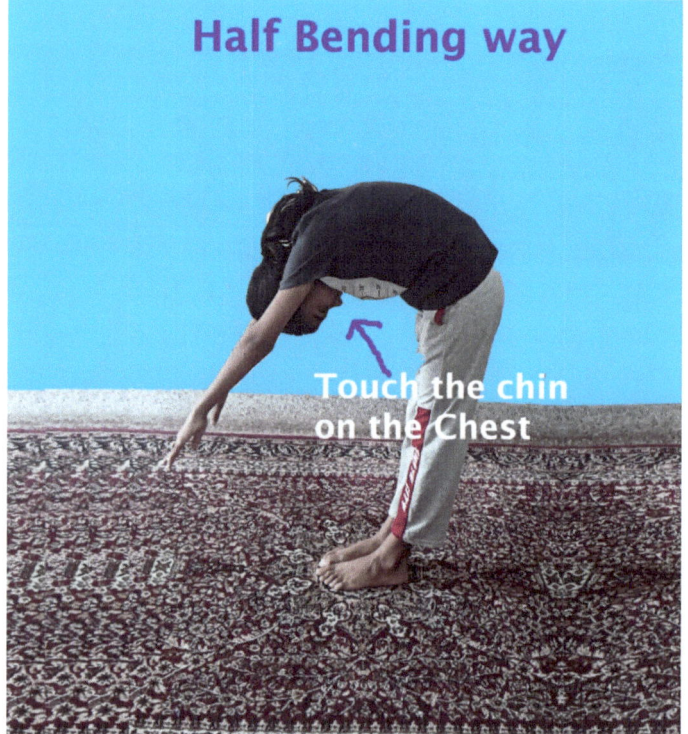

Picture 2: Head Bending and Chin Touching the Chest

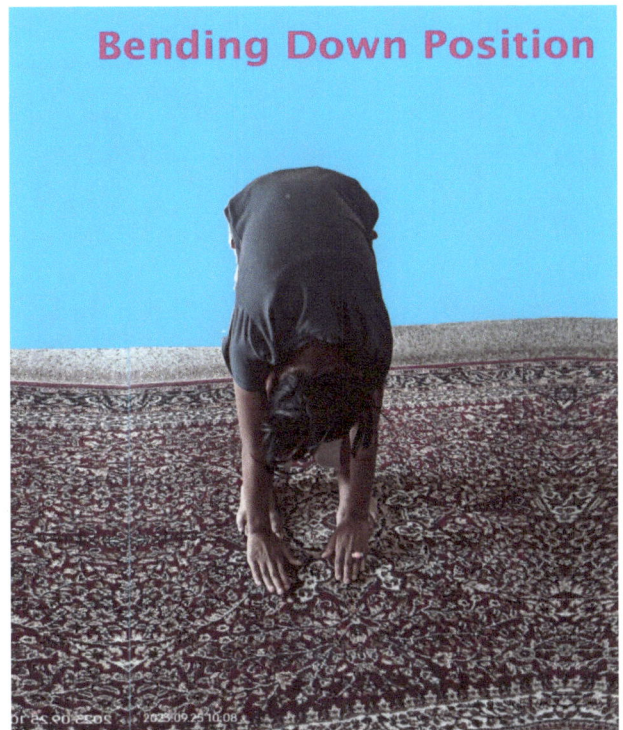

Picture 3: Body Bending and Hands Touching the Floor

Don'ts:

☐ Don't overstretch or stress your body to touch the floor.

Note: After this exercise, drink warm water to aid your bowel movements.

Variations:

- It is possible to carry out step 1 and step 2 as separate activities.
- Depending on your time availability, you can perform them individually or together.

Benefits:

❖ This is one of the balancing exercises.

❖   Embarking on this routine first thing in the morning can help alleviate any stress on the spine from sleep, while simultaneously providing a comprehensive stretch to the entire back.

❖   This posture facilitates proper breathing, additionally enhancing and strengthening the thighs and knees.

❖ It fortifies the colon, aids the digestive process, and promotes regular bowel movements.

❖ It is an ideal practice for *overcoming constipation*.

❖   It is beneficial for managing fevers, headaches, colds, and loose motions due to weather changes.

IV EXERCISE 2: SIT UPS - BRAIN YOGA

"I don't count my sit-ups. I only start counting when it hurts because they're the only ones that count."

-Muhammad Ali

This exercise is presently referred to as brain yoga, yet in India, it has been a tradition since ancient times—a means of expressing gratitude to God. During my primary school days, teachers recommended this exercise to students who sought improvement in their studies.

Technique:
- This is a combination of sitting and standing poses.
- It includes observing the breath.
- Holding ears is part of a therapy

Directions:
- ✓ This exercise can be performed at any time of the day when a revitalizing break is desired.
- ✓ Engaging in it during the early morning proves beneficial for brain activation.
- ✓ Other times, this helps with blood flow and stretching of the body muscles.

Execution of steps:
- ➢ **Stand erect**, keeping feet shoulder-width apart.
- ➢ Position one leg slightly **in front of the other**.
- ➢ Hold your right ear with your left hand and your left ear with your right hand.
- ➢ Ensure that your thumb is positioned in front of

the earlobe, with the fingernail facing outward, and the index finger resting behind it.

➢ **Exhale and descend into a squatting position**, making sure both feet are firmly touching the ground.

➢ Pause for a few seconds.

➢ **Inhale and stand up**.

➢ Alternate the positioning of your legs, with the other leg now slightly in front.

➢ Repeat the sequence of sitting down and standing up.

➢ **Relax**.

Dos:

➢ Perform the movements slowly.

➢ Both feet should be flat on the ground.

➢ If you experience pain, widen the distance between your feet, gradually bringing them closer once you find comfort in the pose.

➢ It may take a few days to achieve the correct pose; strive for daily improvement.

➢ Repeat this routine at least three times, and for optimal benefits, increase repetitions up to nine times.

Don'ts:

❖ Please don't overdo it; this may lead to thigh pain. (If the discomfort persists, continue daily workouts with fewer repetitions; it will help the muscles return to a normal state gradually.)

Variations:

✓ This exercise can be performed with legs together or

shoulder-width apart.
- ✓ Additionally, it can be performed with legs aligned in a straight line or with one leg in front of the other.
- ✓ Another variation involves keeping your legs crossed during the exercise.

- ✓ Following this exercise, it is beneficial to do a simple head massage.

Benefits:

- ➢ This is one of the most powerful brain yoga exercises.
- ➢ It activates brain cells.
- ➢ This exercise refreshes both the mind and body and acts as a stress reliever.
- ➢ It proves helpful in addressing lower-mind states such as uneasiness, sadness, and mental fog.
- ➢ This exercise enhances concentration.
- ➢ It contributes to weight reduction.
- ➢ It harmonizes the respiratory system.
- ➢ It enhances the digestive system.
- ➢ Additionally, it facilitates a quicker connection with the subconscious mind.

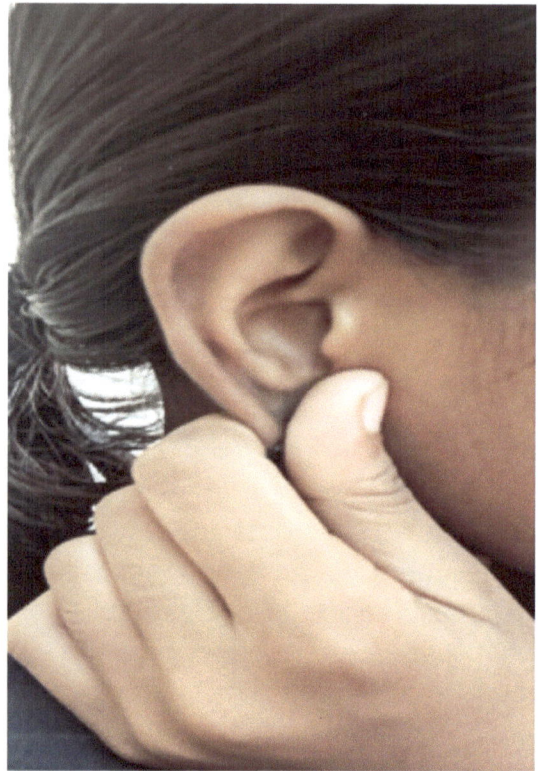

Picture 4: Holding the ear lobe with the thumb and index fingers

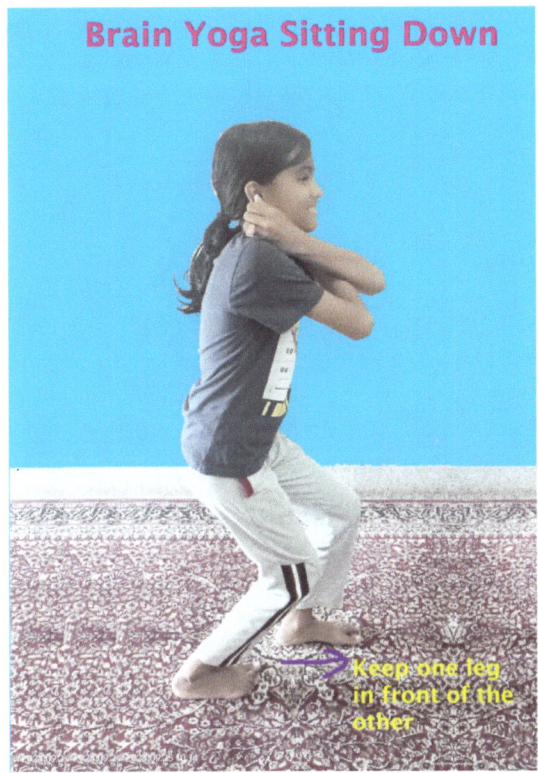

Picture 5: While sitting - halfway.
Keep your legs shoulder-width apart,
with one leg in front of the other.
Hands are crossed, holding the
earlobe on the opposite side.

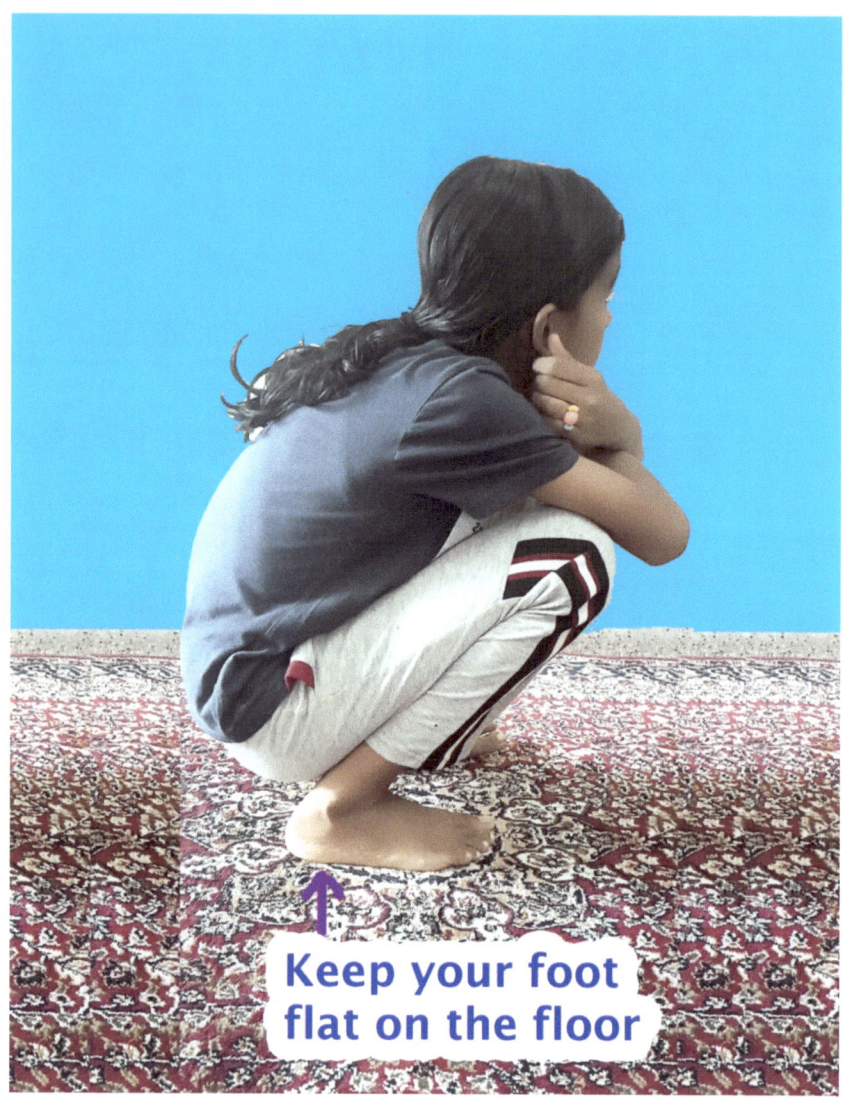

Picture 6: Brain Yoga-Sitting Position

V EXERCISE 3: STYLE WALK

"Go the extra mile. It's never crowded."

- Wayne Walter Dyer

This exercise revolves around the alignment of the body and mind. Walk with your unique style and a sense of enjoyment.

Relish the freshness that permeates your being throughout this exercise, from head to toe. Take note of the sparkle in your eyes.

Prerequisites:

- Keep your chest and shoulders straight.
- Breathe naturally.
- Wear a big smile!

Technique:

This is a combination of:

- Walking,
- Stretching,
- Breathing, and
- Balancing.

Execution of steps:

Step 1: Standing Pose

➤ **Stand straight**, keeping your shoulders straight, with your feet shoulder-width apart.

➤ **Turn your feet inwards at the big toe side** towards the other leg so the small toe side is perpendicular to your body.

➤ When your feet are perpendicular to your body, you should feel a correction in your waist, promoting an upright posture and lifting your chest.

➢ **Keep your knees relaxed**, bending them slightly, ensuring that the body's weight is directed towards the floor rather than the knees.

➢ This position opens up your chest, allowing increased oxygen intake through breathing.

➢ Maintaining this leg pose and body posture, proceed to the next step.

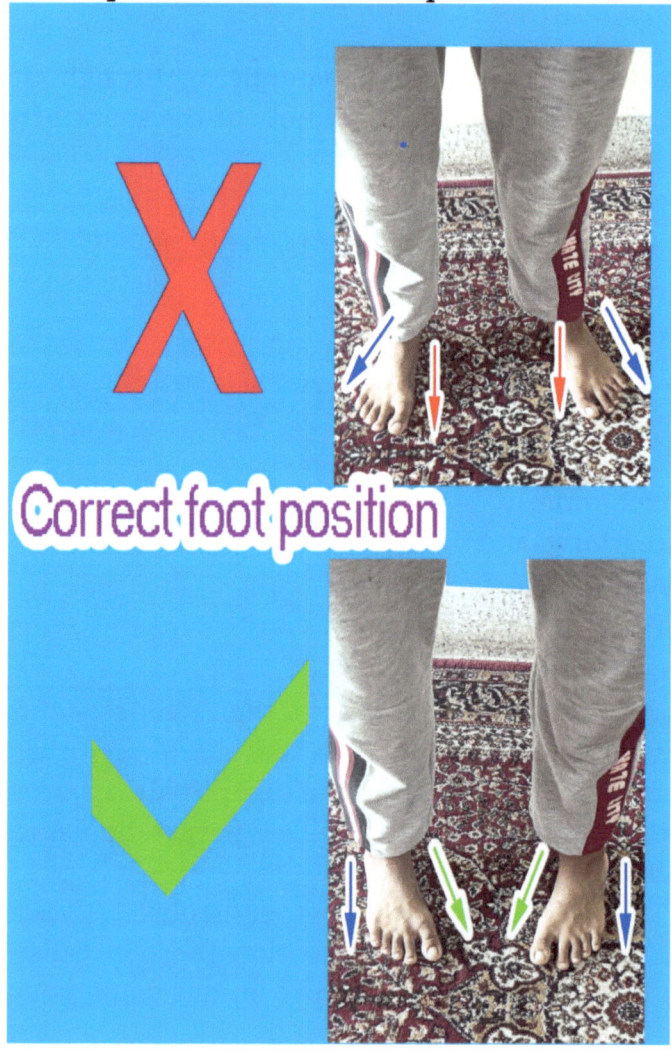

Correct foot position

Picture 7: Standing pose-
Correct position of feet

Step 2: Walking Pose

➢ **Start walking**.

➢ During the walk, ensure that the heel of the bending leg touches or lightly taps your seat, specifically the area at the back of your buttocks.

➢ Keep the non-lifting leg on the ground with the small finger side of your foot perpendicular to your body.

➢ Consciously feel your breath reaching the bottom of your stomach.

➢ Allow your hands and body to sway naturally, infusing your walking style with personal flair.

➢ Embrace the joyous sensation as your body strolls along the metaphorical "red carpet!"

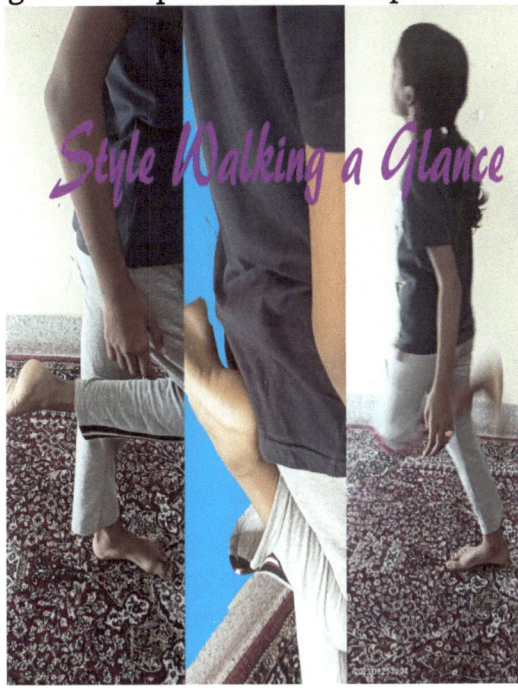

Picture 8: Style walking -
Touching the back and walking pose

Dos:

✓ Maintain an upright body posture, keeping the joints loose at the knees, allowing the body weight to naturally drop towards the floor.
✓ Ensure your movements follow a straight line.
✓ Observe the flow of breath while inhaling and exhaling.

Don'ts:

☐ Avoid bending your back during the walk.
☐ There is no need to consciously control your breath; simply observe the natural flow of inhalation and exhalation.

Variations:

· This exercise can be performed at any time of the day, offering a refreshing break whenever needed.
· This can be performed while:
· Walking,
· Walking in one place, or
· Standing in one place.
· Adopt your "red carpet" style by incorporating movements such as swinging your hands, tilting your body, and inclining your neck.

Benefits:

❖ This is a confidence booster for everyone. So incorporate it as often as possible.
❖ It helps to elongate the chest and lungs.
❖ Elongating the chest expands the front body, particularly the heart and lung regions. This,

in turn, trains the breathing muscles, promoting better oxygen consumption, and contributing to the health of cells.

❖ Enhanced air intake, prana, and life force energy strengthen the respiratory system.

❖ This exercise also contributes to enhancing the presence of the mind.

❖ It facilitates the descent of breath to the bottom of the stomach.

❖ It also promotes the circulation of blood to various parts of the body.

❖ Moreover, it supports our brain cells and improves concentration.

❖ Overall, it balances both body and mind.

VI EXERCISE 4: LAUGHTER ELECTRIFICATION

"You don't have to be good to start; you
just have to start to be good."

— Joe Sabah

Our body generates electricity that flows through it. Similarly, our body possesses its magnetic fields. The human heart creates an electric flow that goes through the body, reaching each cell. This electric flow produces an electromagnetic field.

In alignment with this concept, our body harbours an electromagnetic force. Every physiological function within our body relies on signal transmission – from the immune system to cell regeneration, waste elimination, the nervous system, the circulatory system, and the interplay between the heart and brain. Every cell inherently knows its purpose and capabilities, as well as how to orchestrate the processes required for their realization.

For our body to function optimally, these signal transmissions must be efficient, so that messages reach their intended destinations accurately. In this manner, the network of cells, muscles, and organs communicates holistically.

Since the human body and each living organism on this planet is an electrical entity composed of charged particles, it adheres to the laws of electromagnetism. While the body's bio-electromagnetic fields are exceptionally low in power, they can be measured using devices such as MEG

(Magneto Encephalo Graphy) and MCG (Magneto Cardio Graphy).

This exercise helps heal the path of the life force by inducing it consciously. The best part is that we can influence it using laughter therapy.

Prerequisites:

- Relax for a few seconds.
- Keep your body loose and flexible.

Techniques:

This exercise is a combination of the following therapies:

- Laughter therapy,
- Electrification, and
- Gibberish meditation.

Execution of steps:

➢ **Stand in a relaxed stance** with your feet shoulder-width apart.

➢ **Allow all your muscles to loosen,** cultivating a sense of relaxation.

➢ **Slowly start jerking and shaking** your hands and legs.

➢ Begin shaking your whole body slowly.

➢ Increase the shaking speed to a medium pace.

➢ **Open your mouth and utter gibberish words** like "ahhhhhhhh" or "anggggggggg," or any other meaningless sounds, allowing them to flow in tandem with the rhythmic body jerks.

➢ For a few seconds, **laugh out loud while maintaining the jerking** movements. Let the laughter emanate from the depths of your stomach.

➢   Increase the speed to the maximum you feel comfortable with.

➢   Continue like this for a few more seconds.

➢   Slow down the shaking speed to a medium pace.

➢   Reduce the pace gradually to a standstill.

➢ **Close your eyes and feel the flow of energy in your body.**

➢   Consciously feel the sensations in your head, shoulders, hands, chest, stomach, sides, back, thighs, knees, legs, and feet. Repeat this sequence several times.

➢   Open your eyes slowly.

Dos:

✓   Open your mouth and breathe as necessary throughout the process.

✓   Vary the speed of shaking, increasing and decreasing it gradually.

✓ Feel the rejuvenation of your energy body.

✓   When shaking the head, maintain a slower speed compared to other body parts.

✓   Exclusively for the head, do this movement slowly. Avoid medium or high speeds.

✓ Do it once a day.

Don'ts:

☐   Don't hold your breath.

☐   Avoid excessively fast body movements that may surpass your control.

☐   Refrain from applying undue pressure to

any specific part of the body. Ensure a state of relaxation, allowing for even distribution of weight throughout.

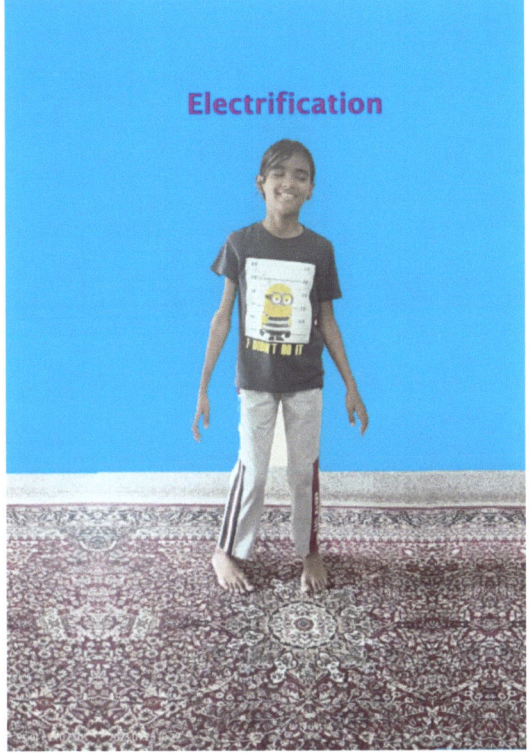

Picture 9: Starting Electrification with less speed

Variations:

- Increase or decrease the pace according to your comfort level.
- This exercise can be performed for the entire body or specific parts, such as hands, legs, etc.

Benefits:

- ❖   The Electrification exercise promotes increased blood flow to all parts of the body.

- ❖ This exercise strengthens the nervous system.
- ❖ It helps to overcome potential blockages.
- ❖ It balances the energy flow of the body.

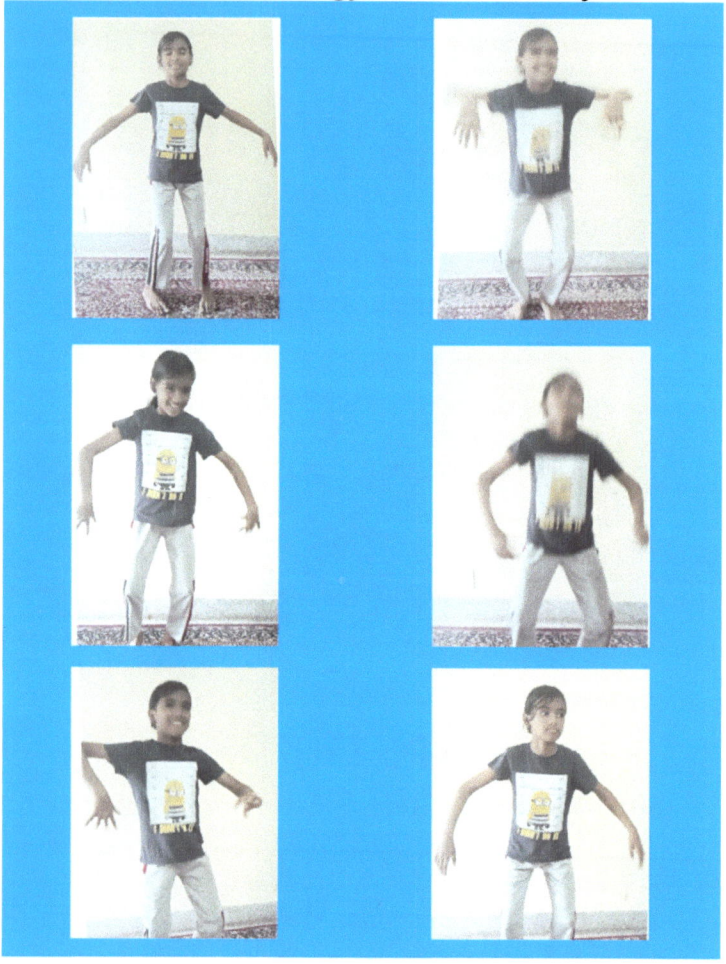

Picture 10: Laughter Electrification in action

VII EXERCISE 5: INFANT YOGA POSE

"Yoga is like a flame that will never dim; the better you practice, the brighter it glows."

— B.K.S Iyengar

Have you ever marvelled at the serene sleeping poses of infants?

Adorable, with their perpetual smiles and constant slumber!

Observe those rosy, chubby cheeks!
They exude an aura of inner tranquillity.
Do these little ones ever shed a tear?
They are reminiscent of a babbling brook!
Often, they maintain a predetermined posture. Could it be their innate yoga pose?
It makes one wonder if we can adopt the same!

I believe it's the Creator's subtle guidance for them to embrace all things healthy. They instinctively follow these cues. As we age, this practice tends to get diluted. Let's partake in their yoga pose for a few minutes.

While this pose appears deceptively simple, it proves to be quite challenging for adults. Achieving this stance requires consistent effort.

It stands as one of the most effective balancing exercises, harmonizing the upper and lower parts of the body. Furthermore, it becomes a straightforward and relaxing pose once we master this relaxation technique.

Technique:

- Assume a simple sleep pose.
- Relax the hands.

- Relax the legs.
- Relax the entire body.

Execution of steps:

➢   **Lie down on your back** in a relaxed and comfortable position.

➢   It is preferable to lie on a mat on the floor rather than on the bed.

➢ **Raise your hands above your head**.

➢ Bend your arms at your elbows.

➢ **Extend your elbows outward**.

➢ Form your hands into **a diamond shape**,

➢ **Bend your legs at your knees** and

➢   **Bring your knees slightly outward** from your body.

➢ Shape your legs into a **diamond form.**

➢ Relax.

Dos:

✓ Observe your body while lying in this pose.

✓ Observe your head, face, neck and shoulders, hands, fingers, chest, stomach, side of the body, back, waist, thighs, knees, legs, ankles, heels, feet, and toes.

✓   Observe the breath flowing down to the bottom of your stomach.

✓ Remain for a maximum of four minutes in this pose.

✓   If drowsiness sets in, return to the regular sleeping pose.

✓   Engage in this exercise gradually, starting with increments of 30 seconds, later progressing to one minute, and so forth.

Don'ts:

☐   Attempting this pose while lying on your stomach

is not recommended.

Variations:

- Perform this exercise either upon waking up or before sleeping, for a brief duration, while lying on the bed. However, it is advisable to do it on the floor to take advantage of flat, solid back support.

- Variations like keeping hands straight or straightening the legs are beneficial.
- While observing your body, try alternating the observation sequence from head to toe and then from toe to head a few times.

Benefits:

- ❖ It enhances relaxation in your shoulders and hands.
- ❖ Energetically, this pose is beneficial for individuals experiencing a sense of confusion.

- ❖ When practised after a long workday or exercise, this resting asana can assist with unwinding and calming the muscles, ensuring a good night's sleep.

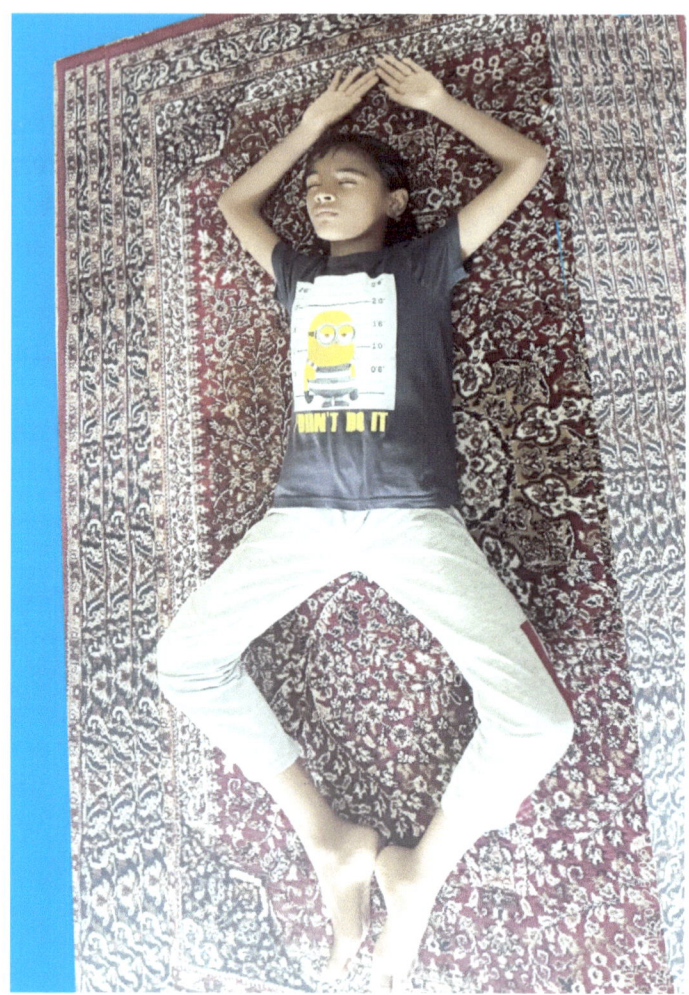

Picture 11: Infant yoga pose

VIII EXERCISE 6: INNER STANCE LIGHT MEDITATION EXERCISE

"Strength does not come from physical capacity. It comes from an indomitable will."

-Mahatma Gandhi

We should dedicate at least five minutes daily to being calm and quiet. This helps to replenish our energy levels, promoting the balance of our systems, and supporting our body's ability to heal. It is all about meditation.

The high frequency of beta brainwaves ranges from 12 Hz to 40 Hz. The more we engage in activities while being influenced by these waves, the more likely we are to experience anxiety, stress arousal, and difficulty relaxing.

The frequency range of alpha brainwaves, which falls between 8 to 12 Hz, is considered moderate. When these brainwaves take precedence, we enter a state of relaxed and passive attention.

Through this meditation, we can anchor ourselves in the present moment. It aids in transitioning from the distractive and 'noisy' beta brainwaves to the calming alpha brainwaves.

This practice supports the calming of the mind, paving the way for connection with the subconscious. In this way, we can align our body, mind, and soul.

This is a meditation technique, complemented by a simple balancing exercise.

Techniques:

- ❖ Sitting calmly.
- ❖ Balancing the body.
- ❖ Neck rotations.
- ❖ Eye coordination.

These techniques are performed simultaneously to get better results.

Execution of steps:

Step 1: Movement of the head

- ➢ **Sit down**, folding your legs comfortably. Sukhasana is recommended.
- ➢ Alternatively, sit on a chair.

- ➢ Rest your hands on your knees.
- ➢ Touch the thumb and index finger, keeping the other fingers straightened (known as Chin Mudra).

- ➢ **Wear a big smile** on your face.
- ➢ Keep your chest and shoulders straight, aligning your spine erect.
- ➢ Start turning your **head as slowly as possible** towards the right.
- ➢ Turn to the extreme right, in line with your right shoulder, and
- ➢ Begin turning towards your left at the same speed as you turned to your right.
- ➢ Extend to the extreme left in line with your left shoulder.
- ➢ Once again, turn towards your right and return your head to the starting position, facing forward.

Step 2: Closing eyes

- ➢ Now **close your eyes as slowly as possible** (take a

minimum of 10 seconds to close the eyes).
➢ **Count slowly from one to ten**.
➢ **Open your eyes at the same speed as you had closed them.**

Step 3: Gratitude

➢ Bring your hands together and touch your palms.
➢ Bend down, allowing your hands to touch the floor.
➢ Say "Gratitude" to all your teachers and gurus, from your childhood until today.

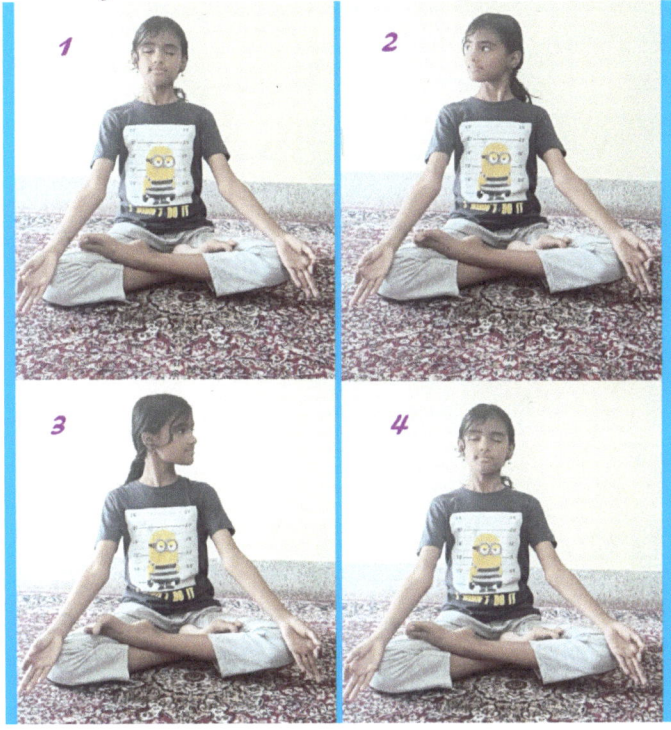

Picture 12: Inner stance light meditation pose

Variations:

■ You can sit in any sitting asana pose.
■ You can stand and perform this.
■ Anyone, anywhere, at any time, can engage in

this meditative exercise.

Benefits:

This technique aids in:

- ❖ Calming down our mind.
- ❖ Improving memory power.
- ❖ Aligning our body and mind with our aura.
- ❖ Building skills to manage our pressure.
- ❖ Expanding self-awareness.
- ❖ Focusing on the present.
- ❖ Enhancing innovation and creativity.
- ❖ Improving tolerance and strength.

IX PROGRAMMING YOUR TIME AND MIND

"Seven days without exercise makes one **WEAK**!!!"

Any workout program you undertake should invigorate both your body and mind. It should not leave you feeling drained. These six super and powerful simple yoga techniques are designed to foster an active, vibrant flow of energy, both physically and mentally.

We have learned the steps of some simple yoga techniques. I hope you find them easy to practice. It is advisable to revisit them repeatedly and gain a good grasp of the techniques.

Some of you, especially those from the '90s, might think, "What's the big deal? They used to be part of our daily lives!"

That is true. These were all part of our daily routines in one way or another, and we didn't notice that they were *the best* workouts for our mind and body.

Indeed, they *were* part of our lives, but as we started turning into robots, living in a more automated world, many of us did not even realize that we had been using them. Let's explore how we can seamlessly integrate these yoga techniques into our daily routines with minimal time and effort. Before delving into our program, let's reminisce about how these practices were an integral part of life until the 80s!

While my emphasis is on India, I presume similar practices have existed in many parts of the globe. People used to get up before sunrise, and after attending to the call of nature (the internal cleansing of our bodies), the first activity would be cleaning the house entrance with a two-foot cleaner or broom (today, a four-foot stick cleaner keeps us at a distance from the floor, limiting the use of joints since we don't need to bend at the waist, knees, or elbows). In those days, people had to bend down and walk in parallel rows, from one end of the hall to the other, to use that cleaner.

Brain yoga (sit-ups or Thoppukaranam) was performed as part of the prayer. Even in schools, it was a practice for slow learners, to enhance their brain functions.

From a young age, children were habitually encouraged to walk with upright chests. It was common for them to carry things on their heads or at the sides of their waists. After working hours, people used to sit under the trees, extending their legs straight in front of their bodies. In a relaxed manner, the legs would fold slightly at the knee, forming a diamond shape. This helped ensure a good flow of blood to the body's organs.

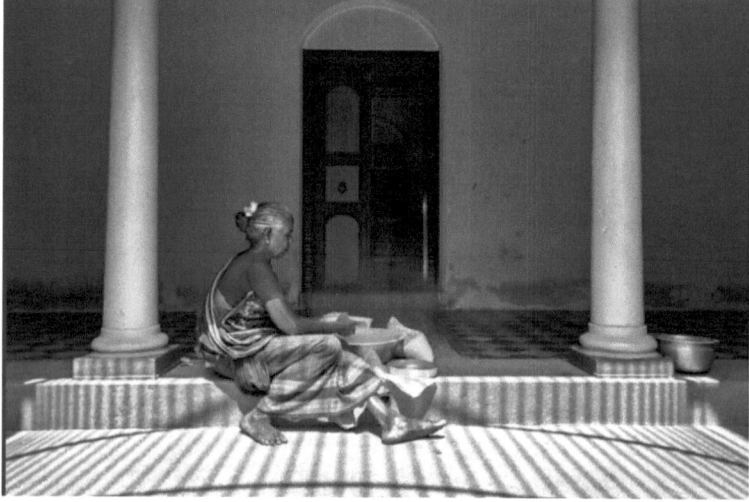

(Picture 13: Image for illustration purposes only; Courtesy:

Internet

During their daily tasks, they would frequently bend down to perform their work, effectively engaging their joints in beneficial exercises.

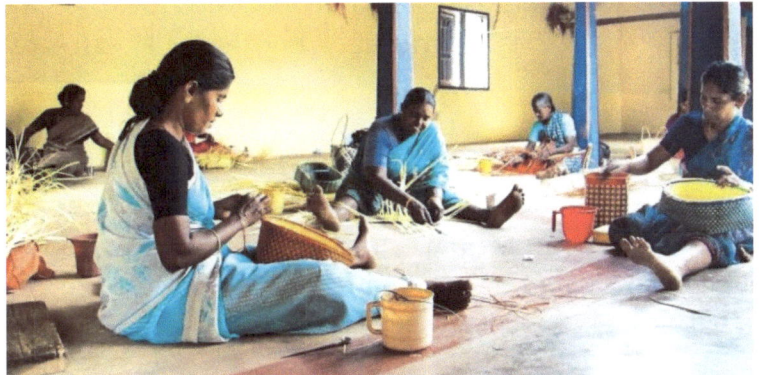

(Picture 14: Image for illustration purposes only; **Courtesy**: Internet)

Now, your mind might think, "Ah, if I could adhere to all of these instructions, why would I ever need to consult this book? It's evident that I would maintain good health." I resonate with your sentiment!

In the "enlightened" robotic world, replicating the same lifestyle pattern may not be simple.

Nonetheless, incorporating essential practices for bodybuilding and healthy living is relatively *easy.*

Here are a few suggestions for seamlessly integrating these six exercises into our daily schedule. They help for effortlessly incorporating these six exercises into our everyday routine.

Program Plan 1: À la carte

Let's assume our typical morning routine involves heading to the bathroom, or brushing our teeth, or at least going to the kitchen to prepare breakfast.

After getting out of bed, engage in Exercise 1 - stretching

and bending.

Do Style Walks to the next destination. Freshen up! Proceed to do the sit-ups.

Now you can begin your daily schedule of activities.

Voilà! Half of the workout program is already accomplished.

At the end of the day, before bedtime, perform the inner stance light meditation and relax with the infant yoga pose.

So far, the electrification part is left out. It is up to you to find a few minutes for the electrification exercise before or after a bath, during tea time, or any free moment. Use it to energize!

Fantastic! The workout is complete.

Program Plan 2: The "Timely Way"

Let's approach this program based on the time factor; let's determine the minimum time required for each exercise so that you can establish a schedule to effortlessly incorporate this program into your daily plan.

The table below outlines the minimum time investment needed.

	Exercise	Time
1	Stretching and bending	1 minute
2	Sit ups	1 minute
3	Style walk	1 minute
4	Electrification	1 minute
5	Infant Yoga pose	1 minute
6	Inner Stance Meditation	2 minutes
	Total	7 minutes

Table 1: The "Timely Way" program plan

One or two minutes are the minimum requirements to perform these yoga techniques. You can choose your preferences and commit to practising them daily.

Program Plan 3: Weekly plan

If you are not prepared to invest seven minutes daily in your health, here is the next plan. Aim to do at least one technique per day. What could be a simpler workout than this? Refer to the day-wise plan below.

	Day	Exercise
1	Monday	Stretching and bending
2	Tuesday	Sit ups
3	Wednesday	Style walk
4	Thursday	Electrification
5	Friday	Infant Yoga Pose
6	Saturday	Inner Stance Meditation
7	Sunday	Holiday

Table 2: Weekly program plan

It is beneficial to alter your workout routine every two weeks to keep your body "guessing" and evolving. When you have the opportunity to engage in your regular workout program, incorporate these exercises. If time is limited, rotate among these six.

To maintain overall health, just one minute for each exercise is sufficient. If weight reduction is your goal, increase the time based on your well-being.

Well, there you have it. Consistently follow the above regimen for six months. While individual results may vary, you will observe progress.

Let's Get Some Self-Motivation

It will require dedication, but imagine the satisfaction you'll feel when you look in the mirror and like what you see. Setting and sticking to goals is crucial, and for good reason.

Everyone has different motivations for needing exercise, and understanding your reasons will help you stay focused on the end goal and your desired outcomes.

If you are like me, you find the journey to good health daunting. Even the path to fitness seems challenging; there are numerous obstacles to overcome, such as health issues, time management, and summoning courage or energy. Whether you've been exercising for a long time or are just starting, new challenges must be overcome. So, how do you put all of this into perspective?

According to Mr. Tom Turner, executive liaison for the Spina Bifida Association, that's precisely where **perspective** comes in. And, according to him,
"There's no mountain too high to climb."
Tom would know. Paralysed from the waist down since birth, he trains thrice a week.
"There are amazing people everywhere doing great things... look around; angels are everywhere! Learn from them."
It is important to learn how to harness the power of your mind to manifest your desires.
Pursuing a routine is much like sowing seeds. You decide what you want to grow and plant the seeds by envisioning and feeling that you have achieved the desired result. You needn't worry about how things will unfold; cultivating the intention with insight will fulfil the purpose. You truly have to remove any weeds you might notice in your path.

When you sow the seeds of your desired outcome in your subconscious mind, your doubts, fears, anxieties, conflicting beliefs, and so on, act as weeds that you need to remove. If you believe that you can't achieve your goal but still want to attempt it, you will eventually quit, and it won't materialize.

Success depends entirely on what you believe is possible for you. Keep in mind that your outer-world experiences only mirror what's in your mind. If you're dissatisfied with your experiences, all you need to do is change your mind about them. Expect only the best in life, express gratitude to your mind and the Universe (God) for giving you the best, and anticipate joyful experiences; your outer-world experiences will reflect this.

Acknowledge that everything in your life forever propels you toward realizing your goals.

Now, why am I sharing all this in the workout program? YES, it does require a significant commitment to allocate 10 minutes daily to your health! Remember, **Health is Wealth!** Daily exercise offers numerous benefits, such as clearing toxins from your body, improving heart health, boosting energy levels, and giving you some rest from mental chatter.

It is commonly thought that slipping up means giving up on your health goals. However, it's important to recognize that everyone fails before succeeding.

Choose an enjoyable activity and diversify your routine. Walk one day, engage in inner stance meditation the next, and incorporate laughter therapy and gibberish during electrification. Design your workout program, commit to it, and strive to achieve it. The possibilities are limitless.

Consider one of Thomas Edison's greatest creations. It's

been said that he made 10,000 attempts before successfully creating a working light bulb. Many might have given up after ten, one hundred, or even 1,000 attempts. Yet, Edison was persistent in his approach. Perhaps he recognized that he needed to discover 9,999 ways not to make a light bulb before reaching his goal. Consider implementing this approach to improving your health and fitness.

X FAQs

"Those who think they have no time
for exercise will eventually have
to make time for **ILLNESS**."

Edward Stanley

What is the optimal time for these exercises?

It is advisable to perform the exercises, or any workouts, on an empty stomach or after a 2-hour gap after consuming a meal. Some exercises can also be done on a per-need basis; please refer to the respective Dos section.

Do I need to follow any particular diet?

It is good to consume a healthy and natural diet. *How* we eat is more important than *what* we eat. Dr. Robert M. Nerem's study on rabbits revealed that social and environmental factors during food intake support good health.

Therefore, maintain a neutral to happy state while eating. There's a saying, "Drink your food and eat your water.

I have an acute illness. Can I follow this program?

In my practice, I have found that acute illnesses like cough, cold, fever, and digestive issues such as loose motions, bloating, etc., can be alleviated with these exercises. Particularly, these exercises are suitable for illnesses caused by weather changes.

What about chronic cases? Can I follow this program if I have chronic issues?

You can incorporate these exercises into your routine if your physician gives you the green light. You are the best judge of your body, so engage in a conversation with it and heed its signals. If you feel comfortable performing these exercises and experience positive sensations, proceed and gradually increase the duration of practice.

They all seem so short and common. Do they really work?

These exercises are simple yet very effective. Our body requires bending or stretching to stay active and healthy. The impulse rate in our body is around 100 meters per second, meaning any impulse created in one body part reaches the other end of the body within 1/100th of a second. Therefore, if a feel-good stretch is done, it only needs a few seconds to bestow its blessings.

Do you have additional questions or require assistance in customizing this program to your specific goals and situation?

Feel free to contact me at: graceprabhamenmai@gmail.com

SUMMARY

"Intelligence & skill can function at
the peak of their capacity when the
body is healthy & strong."

JFK

Our muscles require stretches, and our joints need to bend. Our mind needs to be present in the moment for us to be healthy and happy. Now, you have everything you need to stay happy and healthy.

I have shared my learnings, experiences, and experiments. It is now up to you to translate your understanding into action. Even taking a single step is a substantial achievement towards good health, so begin with that one exercise. You can easily incorporate these exercises into your daily work routine in various ways and forms, improving your overall health.

Just as eating, bathing, and sleeping are crucial for physical and mental health, using our body parts is equally vital. Therefore, performing our tasks independently whenever and wherever possible is preferable to seeking support services. At least these minimum levels of exercise are essential for the body. This is why I named them the "SPS" yoga techniques – Super Powerful Simple.

I have mentioned only some of the primary benefits of these exercises. There are many deep-rooted benefits, which I leave to the readers to experience themselves. These six SPS health yoga techniques are, in fact, a journey towards drugless therapy. It is free medicine or a medication-free path.

So buckle up to take charge of your health and embark on a healthy journey.

Vaazhga Valamudan — Long live, with all the richness of life!

Acknowledgments

I give thanks to the Divine Universe for granting me this incredible opportunity to be an author.

Developing a concept into a book is not easy. The experience is both challenging and rewarding. A word of appreciation is like a world of strength in a time of need. I have received continuous support and encouragement from my family – parents, husband, daughters, friends, and mentors. I am here because of you, and I thank you all.

I especially want to thank my dear daughters, Michele and Suzanne, for their unwavering support in every possible way. Suzanne readily accepted being a model for the yoga poses, and I extend my loving thanks to you, my dear! Michele contributed in various ways, from time management to grammar corrections. My heartfelt gratitude goes to you too, my dear!

I express my sincere gratitude to Mr. Faris for graciously dedicating his time amidst his busy schedule to provide invaluable editing support in short span of time, significantly enhancing the quality of this book. Thank you, Faris.

Special thanks go to my LMNT Neurotherapy guru, Dr. Raman from Ooty, and my yoga guru, Mr. Bapu Kumaran from Guruvayur, for their motivation and selfless teaching that have shaped me into a serious therapist.

My thanks also go to Mr. Healer Baskar and Mr. Gnanasekaran Iya for their selfless teachings on health and lifestyle. I've gained valuable insights from their programs, incorporating them into my own.

I want to express my gratitude to EVERYONE who has ever encouraged me or shared knowledge with me. I listened to every piece of advice, and it has all been meaningful on my journey.

My GRATITUDE and heartfelt thanks to you, my readers, for taking the time to read

"FREE MEDICINE - 6 Super Powerful Simple Health Yoga Techniques"

to help you live a healthy life. I genuinely believe that you now have significant actionable health exercises that will positively impact your everyday life and help you stay healthy and positive.

Could You Please Show Your Appreciation?

May I request one minute more of your time?

If you have enjoyed this book, please consider showing your appreciation by rating and reviewing "*FREE MEDICINE - 6 Super Powerful Simple Health Yoga Techniques*" on Amazon.

Reviews, ratings, and shares are a source of immense support for authors. They are a huge help for budding authors like myself, who aspire to reach a billion followers. Your review will encourage many to practice these exercises and live happy and healthy lives.

Love you all,

Grace Prabha

Return Gift!

I have created a special Telegram channel for the readers of this book who have reached this far, as a note of thanks for your time and effort. I invite you to join my Telegram channel, where I share health tips periodically. Only channel members will be able to join the discussion group to find answers to all their health queries. I will be sharing therapy tips for acute health and mental issues. Please join the channel using the following link.

"Online Health Consultation - Alternative Therapy Methods"

You are welcome to get in touch with me.

@GracePrabhaMenmai
www.graceprabhamenmai.in

My Way of Holistic Therapy

My holistic therapy solutions include:

- LMNT Neurotherapy
- Dr. Bach Flower Therapy
- Acupuncture
- Traditional Energy Medicine
- Electrohomeopathy
- Reiki healing
- Quantum Healing, and
- Counselling

Some of the benefits of the above therapies and remedies are:

- Treating acute and chronic health issues,
- Discovering your 'Inner Self,'
- Gaining clarity about what you want in life,
- Setting achievable goals,
- Making empowering decisions,
- Finding a person's "blind spots", healing them, and growing as a person.

Over the past few years, alternative therapies have emerged as one of the most effective means to create positive changes and lasting results for a healthy life.If anyone requires therapies or like to learn more about the treatments I offer, please feel free to contact me at:

GracePrabhaMenmai@gmail.com

www.ingramcontent.com/pod-product-compliance
Lightning Source LLC
Chambersburg PA
CBHW050815290526
45792CB00001B/126